V. ECHEVERRIA

Top 50 Mat Pilates Workouts

Build Core Strength and Improve Posture with Simple Home Routines

This book was professionally typeset on Reedsy.
Find out more at reedsy.com

Contents

Introduction

Welcome to "Top 50 Mat Pilates Workouts: Build Core Strength and Improve Posture with Simple Home Routines," a guide specially crafted to help you, the reader, embark on a rejuvenating journey towards better health and fitness from the comfort of your home. Whether you're a newcomer to Pilates or seeking to deepen your practice, this book is designed with you in mind.

Structured for simplicity and ease, this book breaks down 50 Mat Pilates exercises that will target all six major muscle groups. Recognizing that everyone's body is unique, each exercise includes modifications to match your fitness level. Additionally, understanding that not everyone may have access to specialized equipment, this book provides creative alternatives using common household items. This ensures that you have the tools to engage effectively with each workout no matter your circumstances. Please consult your doctor or healthcare professional before practicing these exercises.

As you progress through this guide you can expect transformative results not just physically, but mentally as well. Pilates isn't just about building strength and improving posture; it's also about enhancing mental awareness and achieving greater inner balance. By the end of your journey with this book, anticipate feeling stronger, more aligned, and empowered with the skills to maintain your new Pilates practice.

Benefits of Incorporating Pilates into Your Daily Routine

Has the thought ever crossed your mind that there might be an approach to exercise that enhances your health without strain or discomfort? Many forms of physical activity, especially high-impact ones, can sometimes feel daunting or unsustainable, especially if you're dealing with joint pain or other physical limitations. Pilates presents a uniquely adaptable approach to fitness that emphasizes gentle movements to strengthen and tone your body while being mindful of its limits. This chapter will explore the profound benefits that Pilates offers, starting with how its low-impact nature is ideal for anyone seeking a joint-friendly workout regimen.

The emphasis on controlled, precise movements in Pilates also means that each exercise is performed with maximum effectiveness. This meticulous attention to technique helps in cultivating not just physical strength but also mental discipline, as the focus required in Pilates trains the mind to be fully engaged in the present moment, enhancing overall mental acuity and concentration.

This combination of mental and physical exercise makes Pilates a workout routine and a lifestyle approach that significantly benefits strength, flexibility, and mental health. As you progress through the routines and exercises outlined in this book, the gradual build-up of strength will not only be visible in your toned physique but also in your improved overall well-being and performance in daily tasks.

Home Pilates Setup Without Professional Equipment

Rolled-up towels as a strap substitute: Towels can replace Pilates straps to aid in leg stretches or increase the range of motion.

A chair as a support for balance: Use a sturdy chair for exercises like leg lifts or standing stretches, providing stability and balance.

Bench substitute: Perform seated exercises or tricep dips using a stable chair instead of a Pilates bench.

Cushions or pillows as a prop for comfort: Use cushions or pillows to support your back or under your head during exercises that require you to lie down, like in leg stretches or other mat work.

Balance challenges: Use a cushion to stand or step on during balance exercises to increase difficulty by creating an unstable surface.

Elevation: Stack books to create height for exercises needing a step or to elevate the hips during exercises like bridges.

Wall for support and resistance: Use a wall for exercises like wall sits or push-ups to provide resistance and support, helping maintain proper form.

<u>Belt or rope as a leg stretch aid</u>: Use a belt or rope to assist in leg stretches similar to how you would use a Pilates ring or strap, helping deepen stretches and maintain alignment.

<u>Water bottles or cans as hand weights</u>: Filled water bottles can be used as makeshift dumbbells for lightweight lifting exercises. Soup cans from your pantry are also good substitutes for arm weights.

<u>Kitchen counter as a barre substitute</u>: Use a kitchen counter as a makeshift ballet barre for exercises that require you to hold onto something for balance and support.

Tips to Read Before You Start

- Start with 5 exercises per day and slowly work up to 15.

- Focus on your form and execute the moves slowly while breathing deeply in unison with your movements. Form is more important than the number of repetitions.

- Some descriptions may reference starting in a tabletop position or bringing your legs to tabletop. A tabletop position is being on your hands and knees with a strong core and flat back. Bringing your legs to the tabletop position means laying on your back with your knees above your hips and your legs parallel to the ground, forming a flat top. Reference pictures below.

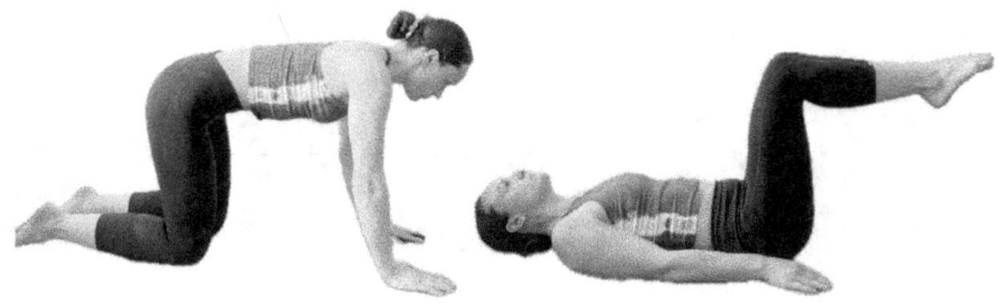

Tabletop Position, Legs in Tabletop

50 Pilates Exercises

1. The Hundred

- Start: Lie on your back with knees bent into your chest, head and shoulders lifted off the mat.
- Action: Extend your legs to a 45-degree angle and pump your arms up and down.
- Repetitions: Inhale for five arm pumps and exhale for five, up to a total of 100 pumps.
- Modifications: Bend knees or place feet on the mat.
- Target Muscle Groups: Core, shoulders, and lungs.

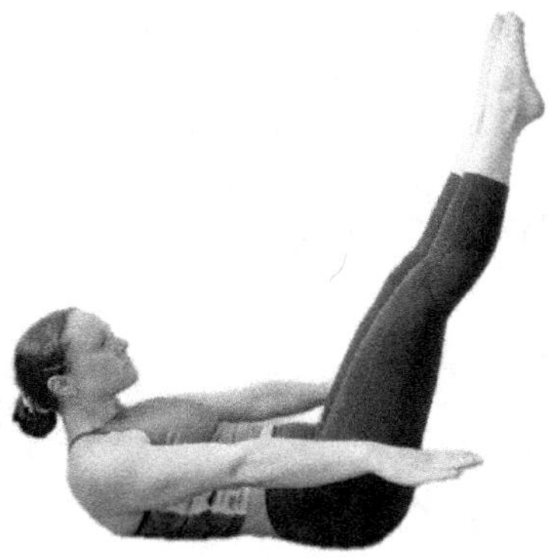

Hundred

2. Roll Up

- Start: Lie flat on your back with your arms extended overhead and legs extended flat on the mat.
- Action: Inhale to lift your arms to the ceiling, exhale as you roll up into a seated "C" curve, reaching towards your toes.
- Repetitions: Perform 5-8 roll-ups. Three sets.
- Modifications: Use a band around your feet for assistance or roll up holding light dumbbells.
- Target Muscle Groups: Core, especially the abdominal muscles.

3. Single Leg Circles

- Start: Lie on your back with one leg extended up toward the ceiling and the other flat on the mat.
- Action: Circle the raised leg across the body and then around in a

controlled manner.
- Repetitions: Do 5-10 circles in each direction per leg. Two sets.
- Modifications: Bend the knee of the raised leg to ease hip tension.
- Target Muscle Groups: Hip flexors, core, and hamstrings.

4. Rolling Like a Ball

- Start: Sit on the mat with knees to your chest, hands on ankles.
- Action: Tuck your chin and roll back to your shoulder blades then roll up, maintaining balance without placing feet on the mat.
- Repetitions: 6-8 rolls.
- Modifications: Hold behind your thighs instead of ankles.
- Target Muscle Groups: Core and spine.

5. Reverse Clam Shell

- Start: Lie on your side with your legs stacked and knees bent at a 90-degree angle. Rest your head on your lower arm, and place your top hand on your hip or the floor for stability.
- Action: Keeping your feet together, lift your top knee away from the bottom knee as high as you can without moving your hips or pelvis. Instead of pausing, continue the motion by lifting the lower leg to meet the top knee. Then slowly lower both knees back together to the starting position.
- Repetitions: Perform 10-12 repetitions on each side.
- Modifications: If you find the full movement challenging, stick to the traditional clam shell by lifting only the top knee and keeping the bottom leg on the ground.
- Target Muscle Groups: Primarily targets the gluteus medius and

minimus on the side of the hip, as well as the core for stabilization.

6. Swimming

- Start: Lie face down with arms and legs extended, head neutral.
- Action: Lift your left arm and right leg, then switch to the right arm and left leg, alternating quickly as if swimming.
- Repetitions: Continue for 30 seconds. Three sets.
- Modifications: Lift only the limbs slightly or one limb at a time.
- Target Muscle Groups: Back, shoulders, glutes, and hamstrings.

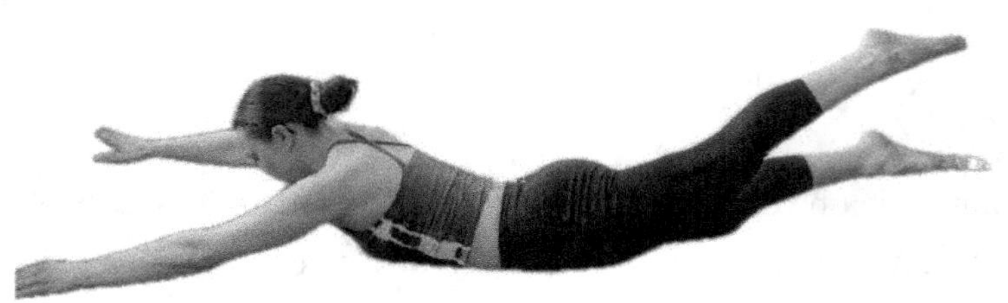

Swimming

7. Marching Standing Up

- Start: Stand tall with your feet hip-width apart and arms at your sides or placed on your hips for balance.
- Action: Lift your right knee towards your chest while keeping your back straight and balancing on your left foot. Lower your right foot gently back to the ground and then lift your left knee. Continue to alternate knees, mimicking a marching motion.
- Repetitions: Continue alternating knees for 20-30 seconds or complete 10-15 lifts per leg.
- Modifications: If balancing is challenging, hold onto a stable chair or counter for support. To increase the difficulty, add a small hop when switching legs or increase the speed of the marching.
- Target Muscle Groups: Primarily targets the hip flexors and core, while also engaging the calves and improving overall balance and coordination.

8. Fire Hydrant

- Start: Position yourself on all fours, similar to the starting position for donkey kicks. Ensure your wrists are directly under your shoulders and knees under your hips.
- Action: Keeping your knee bent, lift one leg out to the side, maintaining the angle at your knee. Lift your leg as high as possible while keeping your hips squared to the ground. Hold briefly at the top, then lower your leg back to the starting position.
- Repetitions: Do 10-12 repetitions on each side. Three sets.
- Modifications: Incorporate a resistance band around your thighs to add difficulty and intensify the workout for your gluteus medius.
- Target Muscle Groups: Gluteus medius and minimus, as well as

your core for stabilization.

9. Open Leg Rocker

- Start: Sit with legs opened wide and held with both hands, balancing on your sit bones.
- Action: Tuck chin towards chest, inhale and roll back, exhale and roll up to balance.
- Repetitions: 6-8 rolls.
- Modifications: Bend knees slightly to maintain balance.
- Target Muscle Groups: Core and balance.

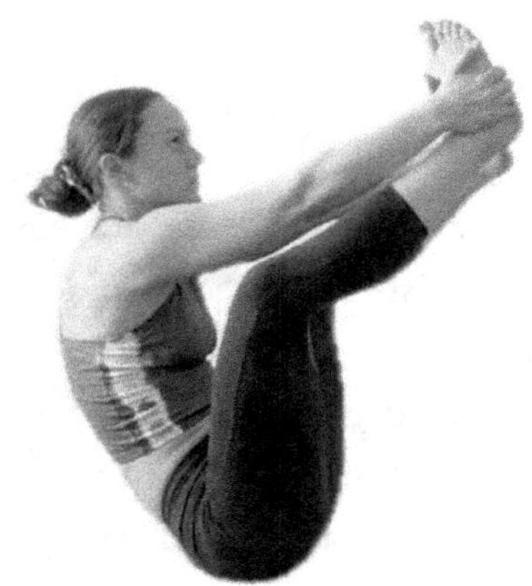

Open Leg Rocker

10. **Corkscrew**

- Start: Lie on your back with legs lifted straight up to the ceiling.
- Action: Circle your legs together to the right, down around, and up to the left, then reverse the circle back to starting point.
- Repetitions: Perform 3-5 circles in each direction. Three sets.
- Modifications: Reduce the range of motion or bend knees.
- Target Muscle Groups: Core, especially obliques.

11. **Hovering Star**

- Start: Begin in a side plank position with your right hand directly under your shoulder and your feet stacked. Extend your left arm towards the ceiling.
- Action: While maintaining the side plank, lift your top leg (left leg) about six inches off the lower leg. Hold this "hovering" position for a few seconds, then lower your leg back to the starting position.
- Repetitions: Perform 5-8 repetitions on each side.
- Modifications: For beginners, start with a modified side plank with the lower knee on the ground to reduce the intensity. To increase difficulty, add a small pulse with the raised leg at the top of the lift.
- Target Muscle Groups: This exercise targets the obliques, shoulders, and glutes. It also engages the entire lateral line of the body for stabilization.

12. **Swan Dive**

- Start: Lie face down, hands under shoulders, legs extended.
- Action: Inhale as you lift your chest off the mat by using your back

muscles, extending your arms and legs straight; exhale as you gently rock forward and back with your body forming a U shape.

- Repetitions: Perform 4-6 dives. Two sets.
- Modifications: Keep your hands on the mat for support if needed.
- Target Muscle Groups: Back extensors, shoulders.

13. Donkey Kicks

- Start: Begin on all fours in a tabletop position, with your hands under your shoulders and your knees under your hips. Keep your spine neutral and your core engaged.
- Action: Lift one leg, keeping the knee bent at 90 degrees, and push your foot towards the ceiling as if you were trying to stamp the ceiling with your foot. Squeeze your glutes at the top of the movement, then return your knee to the starting position without touching the ground.
- Repetitions: Perform 12-15 kicks on one leg, then switch to the other leg. Three sets.
- Modifications: Add a resistance band around your thighs just above your knees or a small weight behind the knee for increased resistance.
- Target Muscle Groups: Glutes, particularly the gluteus maximus, and hamstrings.

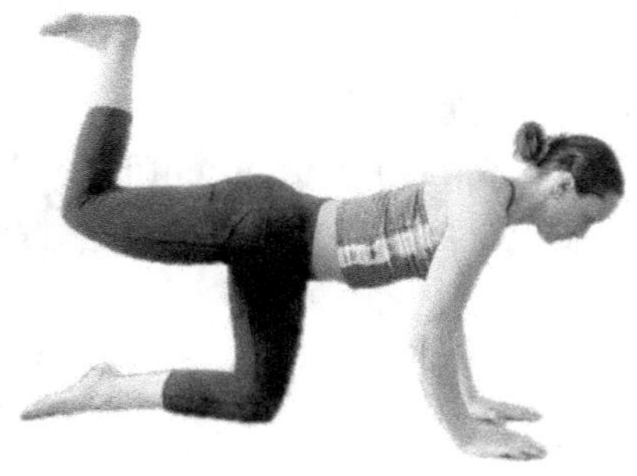

Donkey Kicks

14. **Double Leg Kick**

- Start: Lie face down, hands clasped behind your back, head turned to one side.
- Action: Kick both heels to your buttocks three times quickly, then extend legs and lift chest, reaching hands towards feet.
- Repetitions: Repeat 6-8 times. Two sets.
- Modifications: Keep your head down to reduce neck strain.
- Target Muscle Groups: Back, hamstrings, glutes.

15. **Neck Pull**

- Start: Sit up tall with legs extended, hands behind head.
- Action: Tuck your chin to your chest and roll down vertebra by

vertebra; then roll up to come up and extend your spine. Sitting up straight, tuck your chin and repeat roll down.

- Repetitions: Perform 5-7 rolls. Two sets.
- Modifications: Use your hands to support your ascent if needed.
- Target Muscle Groups: Core, especially the abdominals, and spine flexibility.

16. **Shoulder Bridge**

- Start: Lie on your back with knees bent, feet flat on the mat, arms at your sides.
- Action: Lift your hips towards the ceiling, then extend one leg straight up; lower and lift the raised leg before switching.
- Repetitions: Do 5-8 lifts per leg. Three sets.
- Modifications: Keep both feet on the mat for a basic bridge for 30 seconds.
- Target Muscle Groups: Glutes, hamstrings, lower back.

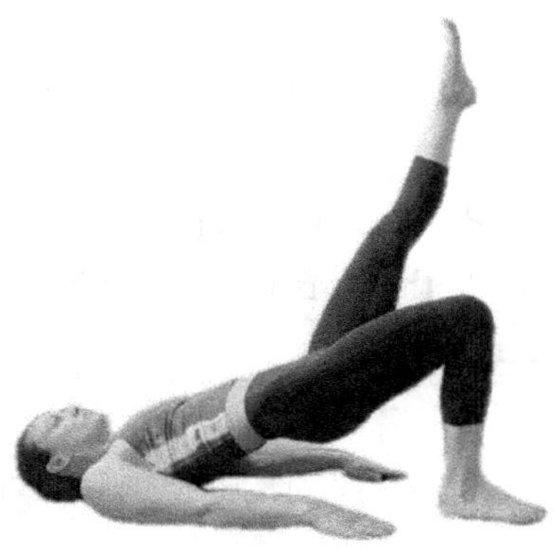

Shoulder Bridge

17. **Arm Circles**

- Start: Sit or stand with your back straight, arms extended to the sides at shoulder height, holding light weights in each hand.
- Action: Make small circles with your arms, the size of a grapefruit, gradually increasing the size of the circles. Keep the movement controlled and smooth.
- Repetitions: Perform 10-12 repetitions in each direction. Two sets.
- Modifications: Decrease the size of the circles if you experience shoulder discomfort.
- Target Muscle Groups: Shoulders, upper back, and arms.

18. **Side Kick**

- Start: Lie on one side, body in a straight line, and prop your head up with your hand.
- Action: Lift the top leg to hip height and kick it twice forward and twice back in a controlled manner.
- Repetitions: Do 10-15 kicks on each side. Two sets.
- Modifications: Perform the kicks with a smaller range of motion.
- Target Muscle Groups: Hip abductors, core.

19. **Teaser**

- Start: Lie on your back with legs in a tabletop position and arms extended overhead.
- Action: Inhale, then exhale as you roll up to a V-sit position, legs extended and arms reaching towards your toes.
- Repetitions: Perform 3-5 teasers.
- Modifications: Keep knees bent or use hands for support behind thighs.
- Target Muscle Groups: Core, especially lower abs.

20. **Bridge**

- Start: Lie on your back with your knees bent and feet flat on the floor, hip-width apart. Arms are by your sides, palms down.
- Action: Exhale and lift your hips towards the ceiling, squeezing your glutes at the top of the movement. Hold for a moment, then inhale as you slowly lower your hips back to the floor.
- Repetitions: Perform 10-15 repetitions. Three sets.
- Modifications: Place a resistance band above your knees to increase the challenge and engage your outer thighs and glutes more

intensively.
- Target Muscle Groups: Glutes, hamstrings, lower back.

21. **Single Leg Kick**

- Start: Lie on your stomach, propped up on your elbows, legs extended.
- Action: Lift one leg so that your thigh is off the ground, bend your knee, and kick the heel towards your buttocks in a quick, small motion twice, then switch legs.
- Repetitions: Alternate legs for a total of 10 kicks each. Three sets.
- Modifications: Perform the kick more slowly if needed.
- Target Muscle Groups: Hamstrings, glutes.

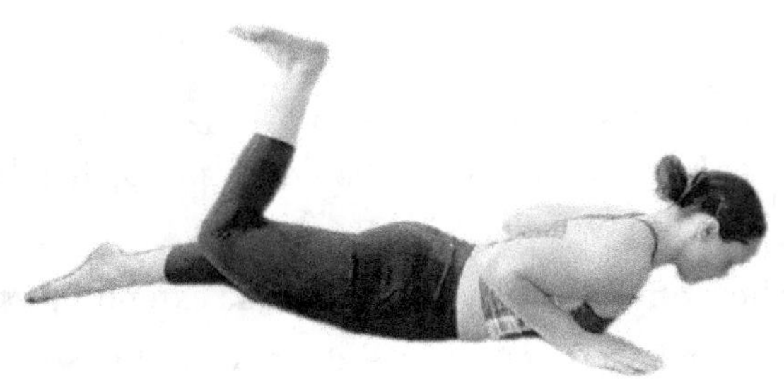

Single Leg Kick

22. **Mountain Climbers**

- Start: Begin in a plank position with your hands placed directly under your shoulders, your body forming a straight line from head to heels.
- Action: Drive one knee towards your chest, then quickly switch and drive the other knee towards your chest, continuing to alternate rapidly. Keep your hips down and your core engaged throughout the movement.
- Repetitions: Continue alternating legs for 20-30 seconds or count each knee drive for a total of 20-30 repetitions per leg.
- Modifications: Slow down the pace of the knee drives or perform the exercise with your hands elevated on a bench or stable platform to reduce the intensity.
- Target Muscle Groups: Core, shoulders, chest, and hip flexors.

23. **Side Bend**

- Start: Sit on one hip with legs slightly bent, top leg in front. Place the bottom hand on the mat under your shoulder, and top hand on your waist.
- Action: Lift your hips off the mat into a side plank, extending your top arm overhead. Hold for 30 seconds. Return to start position.
- Repetitions: Perform 6-8 bends on each side.
- Modifications: Perform with knees bent and resting on the mat.
- Target Muscle Groups: Obliques, shoulders, hips.

24. **Plank**

- Start: Start in a push-up position, with your hands under your shoulders and legs extended back.
- Action: Hold the position, keeping your body in a straight line from head to heels.
- Repetitions: Hold for 30-60 seconds.
- Modifications: Drop to your knees to lessen the intensity.
- Target Muscle Groups: Core, shoulders, arms.

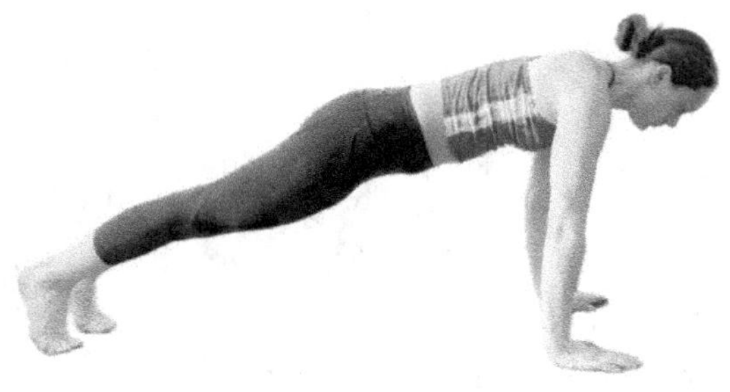

Plank

25. **Pelvic Tuck**

- Start: Lie on your back with your knees bent and feet flat on the floor, hip-width apart. Place your arms by your sides with palms facing down.
- Action: Engage your core and pelvic floor muscles as you slowly

tilt your pelvis towards your belly button, flattening your lower back against the floor. Hold this tuck for a few seconds, then slowly release back to the neutral spine position.

- Repetitions: Perform 10-15 repetitions.
- Modifications: To increase the challenge, lift your hips off the floor into a bridge position while maintaining the pelvic tuck. Alternatively, for those with lower back discomfort, perform the exercise with a smaller range of motion.
- Target Muscle Groups: Core, specifically the lower abdominals and pelvic floor muscles.

26. **Seated Leg Lifts**

- Start: Sit upright in a chair with your feet flat on the floor, hip-width apart. Keep your back straight and place your hands on the sides of the chair for support.
- Action: Engage your core and lift one leg off the floor, extending it straight out in front of you at knee height. Hold the position for a few seconds, then slowly lower your leg back down without touching the floor and lift again.
- Repetitions: Perform 10-15 lifts on one leg, then switch to the other leg.
- Modifications: For less intensity, perform the lift with a bent knee, raising your knee to your chest instead. To increase the challenge, add a pause at the top of the lift or strap on an ankle weight.
- Target Muscle Groups: Primarily targets the quadriceps and hip flexors, with core engagement for stability.

27. **Squat with Heel Lift**

- Start: Stand with feet hip-width apart, arms on your hips for balance.
- Action: Lower into a squat position. Once in the squat, lift your left heel off the floor, balancing on the ball of your foot. Perform squats with the heel lifted and then bring the foot down and repeat with the right heel lifted.
- Repetitions: Perform 8-10 repetitions on each side.
- Modifications: Do not squat as deep if you experience any discomfort in your knees or back.
- Target Muscle Groups: Quads, glutes, calves, and core.

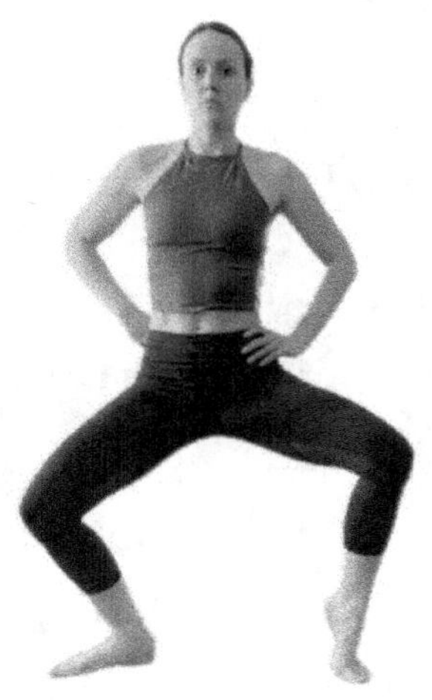

Squat w/ Heel Lift

28. **Push-Up Walk**

- Start: Stand with feet together, roll down to touch the floor, and walk hands out to a plank position.
- Action: Perform a push-up, then walk hands back towards feet and roll up to standing.
- Repetitions: Do 3-5 repetitions. Three sets.
- Modifications: Perform push-up on knees.
- Target Muscle Groups: Chest, arms, core.

29. **Pilates V-Position Heel Raises**

- Start: Stand upright with your heels together and toes apart, creating a "V" shape with your feet. Balance your weight on the balls of your feet.
- Action: Slowly lift your heels off the ground, rising onto the balls of your feet. Hold for a moment, then slowly lower your heels back down.
- Repetitions: Do 10-12 repetitions. Three sets.
- Modifications: Hold onto a chair or wall for balance if needed.
- Target Muscle Groups: Calves, ankles, and core.

30. **Single Leg Stretch**

- Start: Lie on your back, knees into chest, head and shoulders lifted off the mat.
- Action: Extend one leg out as you pull the other knee closer, switch legs.
- Repetitions: Alternate legs for 10-12 times each. Three sets.

- Modifications: Keep head down if neck strain occurs.
- Target Muscle Groups: Core, particularly lower abdominals.

31. **Double Leg Stretch**

- Start: Lie on your back with your knees pulled into your chest, head and shoulders lifted off the floor.
- Action: Inhale and extend your arms and legs outward into a "V" shape, then exhale and circle your arms as you draw your knees back into your chest.
- Repetitions: Perform 8-10 repetitions. Three sets.
- Modifications: Extend legs less or higher towards the ceiling to reduce strain.
- Target Muscle Groups: Core, particularly the deep abdominals.

32. **Single Leg Extension**

- Start: Begin on all fours in a tabletop position with your hands directly under your shoulders and your knees under your hips. Keep your spine neutral and your core engaged.
- Action: Slowly extend your right leg straight behind you, keeping your toes pointed and your leg in line with your body. Hold the position for a few seconds, ensuring your hips remain square to the ground. Slowly lower your extended leg to tap the floor, then lift and repeat.
- Repetitions: Perform 10-12 extensions with the right leg, then switch to the left leg. Two sets.
- Modifications: For added stability, perform this exercise near a wall and use it to help maintain balance if needed.

- Target Muscle Groups: Glutes, lower back, and hamstrings.

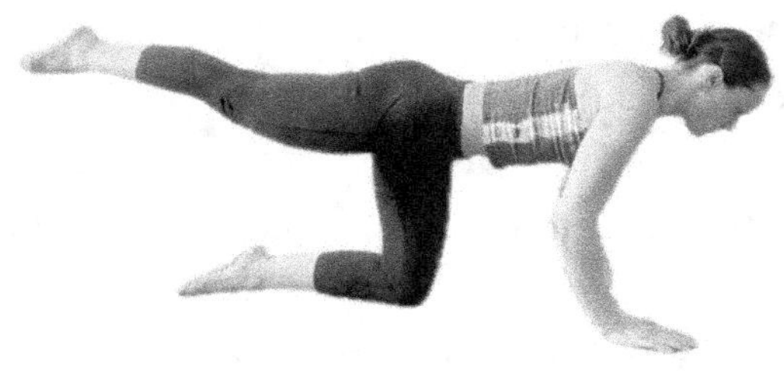

Single Leg Extension

33. **Scissor Switch**

- Start: Lie flat on your back on a mat, with your arms by your sides. Lift your legs to a 90-degree angle from your hips, keeping them straight.
- Action: Lower one leg toward the mat while keeping the other leg raised. Just before your lowering leg touches the mat, cross it over the other leg. Switch the positions of your legs by lifting the lower leg up and lowering the other, crossing it underneath the lifted leg this time. Continue alternating in a smooth, controlled motion, crossing over and under with each switch.
- Repetitions: Perform 10-12 switches for each leg. Three sets.
- Modifications: To decrease the intensity, bend your knees slightly

during the exercise or perform it with your head and shoulders relaxed on the mat. To increase the challenge, keep your legs straighter and lower them closer to the ground with each switch.

- Target Muscle Groups: Targets the lower abdominals, hip flexors, and enhances coordination.

34. **Lower Lift**

- Start: Lie on your back with your legs straight up towards the ceiling and hands under your hips for support.
- Action: Lower your legs slowly down towards the floor, then lift them back up.
- Repetitions: Do 8-10 repetitions.
- Modifications: Lower the legs only partially to maintain control and protect the lower back.
- Target Muscle Groups: Lower abdominals.

35. **Arm Extension**

- Start: Stand with your feet hip-width apart, knees slightly bent. Lean forward at the waist. Hold a lightweight in each hand with straight arms at your sides.
- Action: Keeping your arms straight, extend your arms straight behind your hips, palms facing each other. Squeeze your arms towards each other, bringing your shoulder blades together then slowly return to the starting position.
- Repetitions: Perform 10-15 repetitions.
- Modifications: If you experience lower back discomfort, perform this exercise while seated on a bench or chair, bending forward

from the waist.
- Target Muscle Groups: Triceps, upper back, and shoulders.

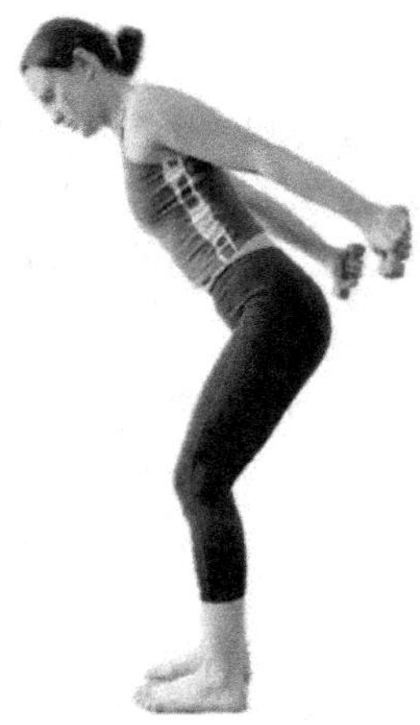

Arm Extension

36. **Saw**

- Start: Sit tall with legs wide apart and arms extended to the sides at shoulder height.
- Action: Twist your torso and reach your right hand towards your left foot, bringing your pinky finger to your pinky toe, then switch sides.
- Repetitions: Alternate sides for 6-8 repetitions each.

- Modifications: Bend knees slightly if hamstrings are tight.
- Target Muscle Groups: Obliques, back, and hamstrings.

37. Hip Twist

- Start: Sit with your hands slightly behind you for support, legs lifted in a tabletop position.
- Action: Rotate your hips to drop your knees to one side, using only your core, lift them back to center and drop to the other side.
- Repetitions: Alternate sides for 8-10 repetitions each. Two sets.
- Modifications: Keep feet on the ground and rotate only the upper body.
- Target Muscle Groups: Obliques and lower back.

38. Banana

- Start: Lie on your side with legs straight and stacked on top of each other, and arms extended overhead. Your body should form a straight line from head to toes.
- Action: Simultaneously lift your legs and upper body off the ground, keeping your arms and legs straight. Your body will form a curved shape, similar to a banana. Hold this position while you engage your core and try to balance on your hip.
- Repetitions: Hold the position for 10-30 seconds, repeat 3 times then switch sides.
- Modifications: For a less intense version, lift only your legs or upper body rather than both at the same time. Alternatively, bend the knees slightly.

- Target Muscle Groups: Core, especially the obliques, and also engages the shoulders, hips, and legs.

39. **Single Leg Pull**

- Start: Lie on your back with one leg extended up and the other leg extended flat on the mat, head lifted off the floor.
- Action: Pull the raised leg towards you twice with both hands, then switch legs.
- Repetitions: Alternate legs for 10-12 times each. Two sets.
- Modifications: Keep the head down or perform with bent knees.
- Target Muscle Groups: Lower abdominals and hip flexors.

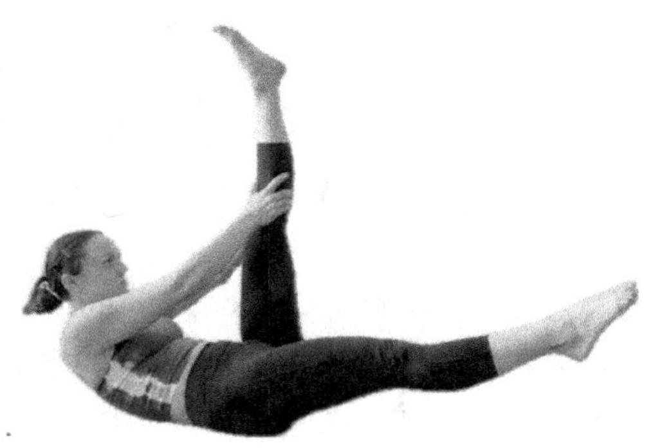

Single Leg Pull

40. **Standing Core Press**

- Start: Stand tall with your feet hip-width apart. Hold a Pilates ball (or a small cushion) with both hands in front of your chest, elbows bent.
- Action: Engage your core and press the ball straight out in front of you until your arms are fully extended, keeping your shoulders down and back relaxed. Hold the extension for a few seconds while continuing to engage your core, then slowly draw the ball back towards your chest.
- Repetitions: Perform 10-15 repetitions. Two sets.
- Modifications: For a less intense workout, perform the exercise without the ball, simply extending your arms. To increase the difficulty, perform the press on one leg to add a balance challenge, or use a heavier weight instead of the ball.
- Target Muscle Groups: Primarily targets the core muscles, especially the transverse abdominis, and also engages the shoulders and upper back.

41. **Pilates Lunge with Twist**

- Start: Stand tall with your feet together and arms raised in front of you at shoulder height.
- Action: Take a step backward with your right foot, landing on the ball of the foot and bending both knees to lower into a lunge. Ensure your left knee is aligned with your left ankle. As you lunge, rotate your upper body to the left, extending your arms out to the sides at shoulder height. Rotate back to center and push off your right foot to return to the starting position.
- Repetitions: Perform 8-10 repetitions on each side. Two sets.

- Modifications: For beginners, perform the lunge without the twist or with a shallower lunge to reduce the strain on the knees. To increase the difficulty, hold a light dumbbell in each hand while performing the twist, or increase the depth of the lunge.
- Target Muscle Groups: This exercise targets the quadriceps, hamstrings, glutes, and core, with an additional focus on the obliques due to the twisting motion.

42. **Rainbow**

- Start: Begin on all fours in a tabletop position with your hands under your shoulders and knees under your hips. Ensure your back is flat and your core is engaged.
- Action: Extend your right leg out to the side, toes pointed. Lift the leg up and arc it over to the opposite side as if drawing a rainbow with your toes. Touch the toes lightly to the ground, then lift and arc the leg back to the starting position on the side.
- Repetitions: Perform 10-12 repetitions on one side, then switch to the other leg. Two sets.
- Modifications: For beginners, decrease the height of the arc or the range of motion. To increase the challenge, add an ankle weight to the working leg or hold the leg for a moment at the top of the arc.
- Target Muscle Groups: Targets the gluteus maximus, gluteus medius, and core muscles.

43. **Heel Lifts in Plank**

- Start: Begin in a plank position with your arms extended under your shoulders, body in a straight line from head to heels.

- Action: While maintaining a strong plank, lift your heels off the ground by pressing onto the balls of your feet, then lower them back down.
- Repetitions: Perform 10-15 repetitions of lifting and lowering your heels. Two sets.
- Modifications: Drop to your knees for a modified plank if maintaining a full plank position is too challenging.
- Target Muscle Groups: Core, calves, and shoulders.

44. **Single Leg Balance with Reach**

- Start: Stand tall with your feet hip-width apart. Shift your weight onto your left foot, and find your balance.
- Action: Slowly lift your right foot off the ground, bending the knee so your right leg is in a 90-degree position. As you balance on your left leg, extend your right arm forward at shoulder height. Hold this position while focusing on maintaining stability. For an added challenge, slowly reach your right arm to the right side, then across your body to the left, moving only your arm while keeping the rest of your body stable.
- Repetitions: Hold the balance for 10-30 seconds, then switch legs and repeat the sequence.
- Modifications: To decrease the difficulty, keep your toe of the lifted leg lightly touching the floor instead of lifting the foot completely. To increase the challenge, close your eyes or stand on a soft surface like a foam mat.
- Target Muscle Groups: This exercise targets the core stabilizers, the glutes and hip stabilizers of the standing leg, and the shoulders and upper back as the arm moves.

45. **Bicycle**

- Start: Lie on your back with hands behind your head and legs in a tabletop position.
- Action: Extend one leg out as if pedaling a bicycle while bringing the opposite elbow to the opposite knee, alternating sides.
- Repetitions: Continue for 12-15 cycles each side. Three sets.
- Modifications: Perform the movement slowly or with higher leg extension to reduce difficulty.
- Target Muscle Groups: Core, especially the obliques.

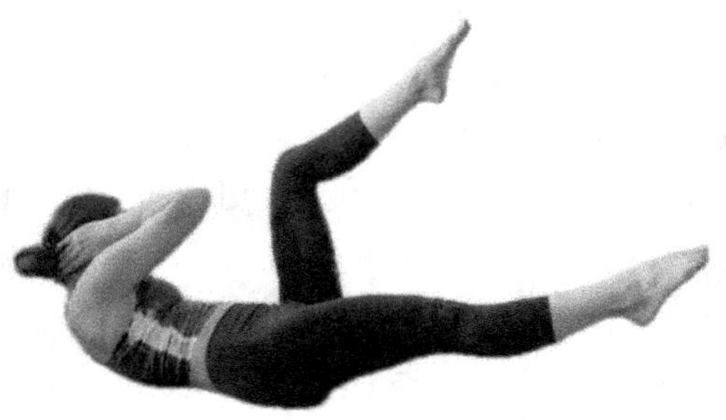

Bicycle

46. **Clam Shell**

- Start: Lie on your side with your hips and knees bent at a 45-degree angle, legs stacked. Rest your head on your lower arm, and place your top hand on your hip.

- Action: Keeping your feet together, raise your upper knee as high as you can without shifting your hips or pelvis. Pause, then slowly lower the knee to the starting position.
- Repetitions: Perform 12-15 repetitions on each side.
- Modifications: Add a resistance band around your thighs just above your knees to increase the difficulty.
- Target Muscle Groups: Glutes, specifically the gluteus medius.

47. Bicep Curls

- Start: Stand or sit with your back straight, arms by your sides, and palms facing forward, holding light weights.
- Action: Curl the weights towards your shoulders by bending your elbows, keeping your upper arms stationary. Slowly lower the weights back down to the starting position.
- Repetitions: Perform 10-12 repetitions. Two sets.
- Modifications: Use lighter weights if the exercise feels too strenuous or if maintaining form becomes challenging.
- Target Muscle Groups: Biceps, forearms.

48. Standing Back Fly

- Start: Stand with your feet hip-width apart and knees slightly bent. Lean forward slightly at your hips, keeping your back flat and core engaged. Arms hang directly under your shoulders with palms facing each other, holding light weights.
- Action: Exhale as you lift both arms out to the sides and slightly

up towards the ceiling, squeezing your shoulder blades together. Your arms should be slightly bent at the elbows. Hold the position briefly at the top of the movement before inhaling as you slowly lower your arms back to the starting position.

- Repetitions: Perform 10-12 repetitions. Two sets.
- Modifications: For a less intense workout, perform the exercise without weights or with very light weights. To increase the challenge, add heavier weights or increase the hold time at the top of the movement.
- Target Muscle Groups: Targets the upper back muscles, particularly the rhomboids and trapezius, as well as engaging the rear deltoids.

49. **Angel Arms**

- Start: Lie on your back with arms by your sides, palms facing up.
- Action: Slowly move your arms in a wide arc over your head and then back down to your sides.
- Repetitions: Perform 10-12 repetitions. Three sets.
- Modifications: Reduce the range of motion if shoulder discomfort occurs.
- Target Muscle Groups: Shoulders, upper back.

50. **Tricep Extensions**

- Start: Stand with feet hip-width apart, a lightweight in one hand. Raise the weight above your head, arm straight, the other hand on your waist.
- Action: Slowly bend your elbow to lower the weight behind your

head, keeping your upper arm close to your ear. Extend your arm back to the starting position.

- Repetitions: Perform 10-12 repetitions, then switch arms. Two sets.
- Modifications: Perform the exercise seated for better stability if standing causes imbalance or discomfort.
- Target Muscle Groups: Triceps, shoulders.

Cooldown

Cat and Cow Stretch

- Start: Start on your hands and knees, with your wrists under your shoulders and knees under your hips.
- Action: Round your back towards the ceiling while tucking your head toward your chest (like a cat). Inhale as you drop your belly towards the mat, lift your chin and chest, and gaze up toward the ceiling, arching your back.
- Repetitions: Flow between Cow and Cat stretches for 8-10 cycles.

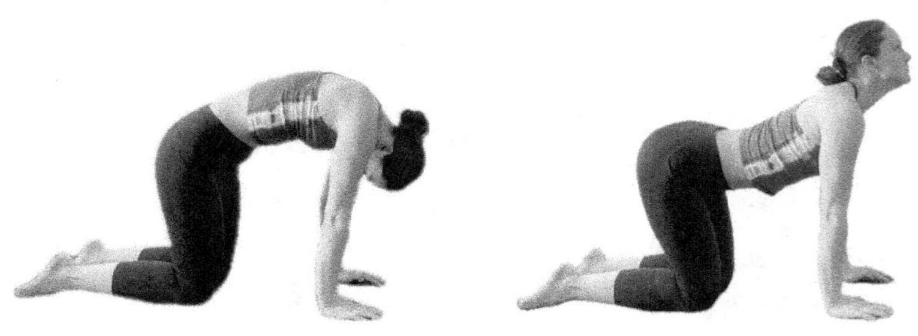

Cat , Cow

Standing Side Split

- Start: Stand with your feet wider than hip-width apart, toes pointing forward.
- Action: Shift your weight to one side, bending one knee while keeping the other leg straight, then switch sides.
- Repetitions: Alternate sides for 8-10 repetitions each.
- Modifications: Decrease the depth of the squat or perform it without any weights.
- Target Muscle Groups: Inner thighs, glutes.

Mermaid Stretch

- Start: Sit with legs folded to one side, one hand on the floor beside you.
- Action: Lift the other arm overhead and bend towards the side with the hand on the floor, stretching the side of your body.
- Repetitions: Stretch each side 3-5 times.
- Modifications: Perform the stretch while seated on a chair.
- Target Muscle Groups: Obliques, latissimus dorsi.

Spine Twist Supine

- Start: Lie on your back with arms extended to the sides at shoulder level and legs lifted in a tabletop position.
- Action: Rotate your legs to one side and extend your top leg while keeping your upper back pressed to the floor, then switch to the other side.
- Repetitions: Alternate sides for 6-8 repetitions each.

- Modifications: Keep the angle of the knees closer to the chest to reduce the rotational load.
- Target Muscle Groups: Obliques and lower back.

Tricep Stretch

- Start: Stand or sit upright with your feet hip-width apart. Raise your right arm straight up over your head.
- Action: Bend your elbow to bring your right hand towards your upper back, palm facing down towards your spine. Use your left hand to gently push back on your right elbow to deepen the stretch. Hold the position and feel the stretch in your right tricep.
- Repetitions: Hold the stretch for 15-30 seconds on each side.
- Modifications: If reaching your elbow is difficult, use a towel or strap to assist the stretch by holding it with both hands.
- Target Muscle Groups: Triceps, shoulders.

Continue Your Journey

Incorporating Pilates into your daily routine can be both enjoyable and highly beneficial for your physical and mental well-being. Start by setting aside a consistent time each day, perhaps in the morning to energize for the day ahead or in the evening to unwind before bed. Even just 10-15 minutes can make a significant difference if you maintain consistency. Additionally, integrate Pilates principles into everyday activities; for instance, practice proper posture while sitting at your desk or engage your core muscles while walking. As Pilates is as much about mindfulness as it is about physical exercise, try to stay present and focused throughout your day and seamlessly blend Pilates into your daily life.

Pilates is more than just a workout—it's a way to enhance your life's quality through improved physical health, mental clarity, and reduced stress. Embrace these practices, and let them transform you from the inside out.